Stop the Allergic Reaction Before It Starts

By Kerri Ryan

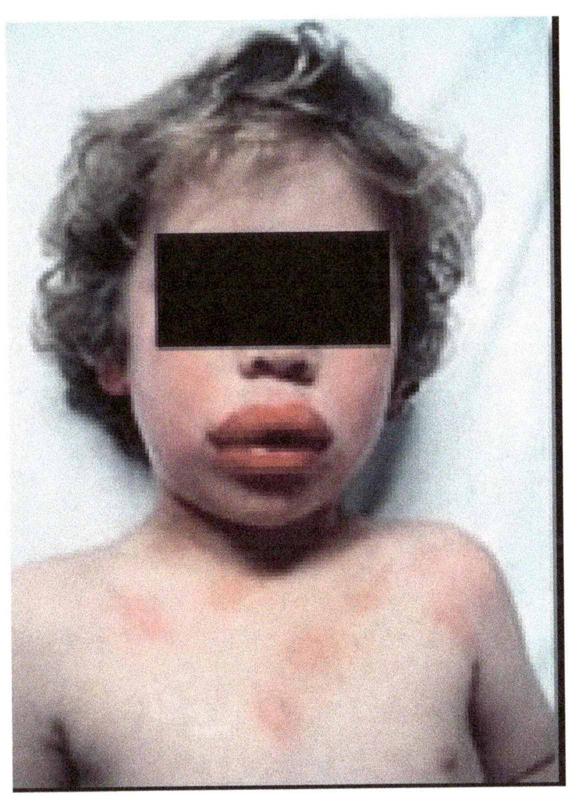

www.Nutritional-Therapy.us

Contents

Allergies on the Rise

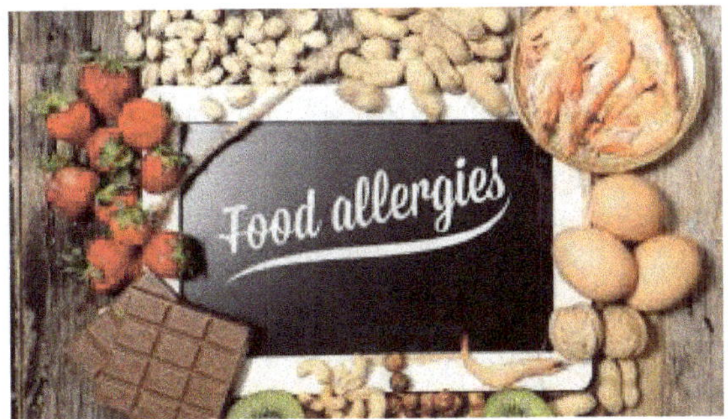

When I was a kid, very few people had allergies. Even then it was only for a few weeks in the Spring when the pollen started to bloom. These days, it is rare to find anyone who doesn't have some allergies of one kind or another. More and more people are being diagnosed with allergies; and at earlier ages than ever before in history. It is not just that we have better methods to track and diagnose them, but insurance claims are way up, with significantly higher numbers of people making routine visits to the doctor for allergy treatments.

This increase is so profound, that our society has actually begun to cater to allergy sufferers on a professional level. There are now daily publications announcing pollen counts, and allergen forecasts to help many plan their day. Hotels have even started promoting premium rooms that are guaranteed to be allergen free for those who simply can't make it through the day without some sort of anti-allergy assistance. These allergen free rooms can cost between $50 and $250 more than a standard room rate simply because there is a market that will support it, and these numbers are climbing all the time. Allergies and their symptoms have become so severe that supporters of the Americans with Disabilities Act (ADA) have successfully lobbied to get allergies classified as a handicap, and listed on the ADA's list of recognized limitations, found in Section 504[1]. Legally speaking, handicapped people are defined as;

> *"...someone who has a physical or mental impairment that substantially limits one or more major life activities, or is regarded as having such impairments."*

Because breathing, eating, working and going to school are "major life activities" asthma and allergies are still considered disabilities under the ADA, even if symptoms are controlled by medication.

A study published in the journal 'Pediatrics' in June of 2011[2] shows that 6 million children, or 2 out of every 8 children counted suffer from food allergies alone. They have found that at least 8% of American children suffer from at least one kind of food allergy, and four out of ten of them will have severe or even fatal reactions. This was far more than was previously believed. The symptoms these kids suffer from will include skin rashes, wheezing, difficult breathing and low blood pressure. These types of health issues were rarely seen before World

War II, and increased in frequency alongside the increased consumption of processed foods. All this-despite all the improved environmentalist interventions and achievements.

While medication has the ability to control the signs and symptoms for allergies, especially in an emergency situation, the body will eventually build up a resistance to these drugs so that sooner or later they will stop working, and leave the patient more susceptible to allergies than they were before. The patient will then have to move on to try something new and typically something with a greater possibility of side effects. What most people are not aware of is that hundreds of allergy medications are recalled every year because of the negative effects of long term use.

In March of 2018[3], Carina Wolff[4] wrote an article titled *7 Unexpected & Potentially Dangerous Side Effects Of Taking Allergy Medicine Long-Term*. Among the issues listed, you will find

Memory Loss   **Diabetes**
Sleep Loss   **Mood Swings**
High Blood Pressure **Osteoporosis**
Vocal Chord
Dysfunction

This news really explains a lot, doesn't it. This is a scary look at just how we are damaging our bodies with meds just because we don't know what else to do. Well, there are alternatives, other ways to recalibrate the bodies systems and cause them to work like they were designed to, however;

Every cause is considered; except the diet.

Like all metabolic diseases, reoccurring allergies will respond to diet and nutrition far better than they will to the synthetic drugs in the long run. Drugs will provide an immediate relief, but only by adding to the diet will sufferers be able to find long term relief or permanent recovery without side effects. Often times these dietary changes are little more than the addition of a few things to the diet and not a completely new menu. Once people understand how their body works, and what it needs to combat a foreign allergen, they can start to build up a resistance to allergens no matter what triggered them, without side effects, and with lasting change.

Billion Dollar a Year Business

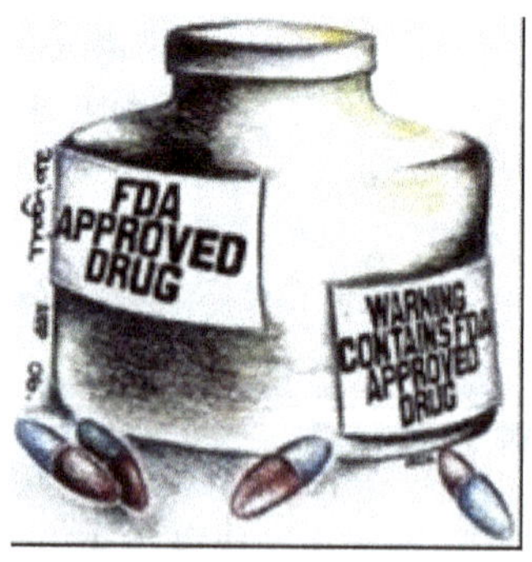

Like many pharmaceutical products, allergy relief is a billion dollar a year business. It is found in every market from the heavily regulated, licensed medical specialist; to an over the counter drug sold in dollar stores. If a product brings relief from allergies there is a market for it, whether it has long term effects or not. Manufacturers will simply print a disclaimer on the box warning users not to use their product for an extended period of time and they continue to profit without fear of reprisals. However, this means little to someone who is up all night coughing, wheezing, and suffering from a pounding headache. They will do almost anything to escape these symptoms, even trade these allergies for some other ailment that is more tolerable.

Anyone in America who goes to open a newspaper, a magazine, or watches TV for an hour or more will sooner or later encounter some sort of prescription drug commercial that promises heavenly deliverance from allergy symptoms. These products are plastered on the side of buses driving through town; thrown at us from the TV and internet several times a day, and free samples are even sent to our homes with the hope of recruiting new customers that will get hooked on a new drug that will make them believe that they just can't live without it. The Truth is allergy medicines will only treat the symptoms, and never solve the real problem. Many doctors will tell you that up front, 'there is no cure for allergies; you may have to stay on these meds for the rest of your life…' and if you continue to take their advice; you will. Most manufacturers understand that many of their products have a limited life span for sale. It is just a matter of time before the long term effects are discovered, and the FDA will rescind its approval.

Miraculously, manufacturers will have by this time come up with a new and improved version ready to enter the market. This cycle plays out daily with one drug after another, all across the country, day after day, year after year while the poor patient only moves from bad to worse with no end in sight. There are those who will try to sell this reality as "progress", part of the process towards finding that perfect drug, but in Truth they are only trading one health issue for another, yet never fully reaching the real goal of being truly healthy. All the while, the pharmaceutical companies continue to rake in billions from this army of willing volunteers who simply don't know what else to do.

<u>U.S. Department of Commerce, How Much of a Markup Drugs Have</u>

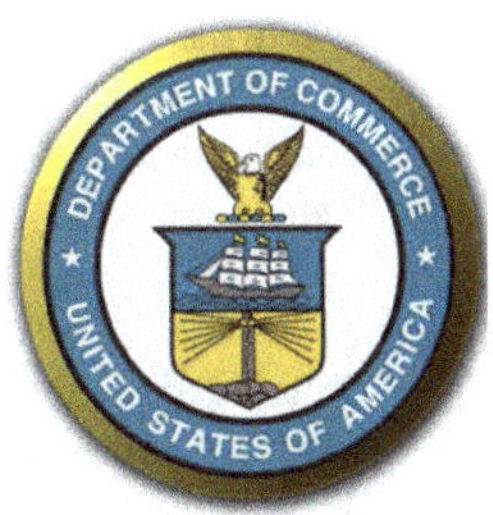

Here is a brief article written by Sharon L. Davis, Budget Analyst, U.S. Department of Commerce, on how much of a markup drugs have in today's world, and just how much money these pharm companies are making. It is no wonder that they run the health care industry.

Let's hear it for Costco!
By Sharon L. Davis, Budget Analyst, U.S. Department of Commerce
Make sure you read all the way past the list of the drugs. The woman that signed below
is a Budget Analyst out of federal Washington, DC offices.
Did you ever wonder how much it costs a drug company for the active ingredient in
prescription medications? Some people think it must cost a lot, since many drugs sell
for more than $2.00 per tablet.
We did a search of offshore chemical synthesizers that supply the active ingredients
found in drugs approved by the FDA. As we have revealed in past issues of Life
Extension, a significant percentage of drugs sold in the United States contain active

ingredients made in other countries. In our independent investigation of how much profit
drug companies really make, we obtained the actual price of active ingredients used in
some of the most popular drugs sold in America. The data below speaks for itself.

Celebrex: 100 mg
Consumer price (100 tablets): $130.27
Cost of general active ingredients: $0.60
Percent markup: 21,712%

Claritin: 10 mg
Consumer Price (100 tablets): $215.17
Cost of general active ingredients: $0.71
Percent markup: 30,306%

Keflex: 250 mg
Consumer Price (100 tablets): $157.39
Cost of general active ingredients: $1.88
Percent markup: 8,372%

Lipitor: 20 mg
Consumer Price (100 tablets): $272.37
Cost of general active ingredients: $5.80
Percent markup: 4,696%

Norvasc: 10 mg
Consumer price (100 tablets): $188.29
Cost of general active ingredients: $0.14
Percent markup: 134,493%

Paxil: 20 mg
Consumer price (100 tablets): $220.27
Cost of general active ingredients: $7.60
Percent markup: 2,898%

Prilosec: 20 mg
Consumer price (100 tablets): $360.97
Cost of general active ingredients $0.52
Percent markup: 69,417%

Prozac: 20 mg
Consumer price (100 tablets) : $247.47
Cost of general active ingredients: $0.11
Percent markup: 224,973%

Tenormin: 50 mg
Consumer price (100 tablets): $104.47
Cost of general active ingredients: $0.13
Percent markup: 80,362%

Vasotec: 10 mg
Consumer price (100 tablets): $102.37
Cost of general active ingredients: $0.20
Percent markup: 51,185%

Xanax: 1 mg
Consumer price (100 tablets) : $136.79
Cost of general active ingredients: $0.024
Percent markup: 569,958%

Zestril: 20 mg
Consumer price (100 tablets) $89.89
Cost of general active ingredients $3.20
Percent markup: 2,809%

Zithromax: 600 mg
Consumer price (100 tablets): $1,482.19
Cost of general active ingredients: $18.78
Percent markup: 7,892%

Zocor: 40 mg
Consumer price (100 tablets): $350.27
Cost of general active ingredients: $8.63
Percent markup: 4,059%

Zoloft: 50 mg
Consumer price: $206.87
Cost of general active ingredients: $1.75
Percent markup: 11,821%

Since the cost of prescription drugs is so outrageous, I thought everyone should know
about this. Please read the following and pass it on. It pays to shop around. This helps
to solve the mystery as to why they can afford to put a Walgreen's on every corner.
On Monday night, Steve Wilson, an investigative reporter for Channel 7 News in Detroit,
did a story on generic drug price gouging by pharmacies. He found in his investigation,
that some of these generic drugs were marked up as much as 3,000% or more. Yes,
that's not a typo: three thousand percent! So often, we blame the drug companies for
the high cost of drugs, and usually rightfully so. But in this case, the fault clearly lies with
the pharmacies themselves. For example, if you had to buy a prescription drug, and
bought the name brand, you might pay $100 for 100 pills.

The pharmacist might tell you that if you get the generic equivalent, they would only cost
$80, making you think you are 'saving' $20. What the pharmacist is not telling you is that
those 100 generic pills may have only cost him $10! At the end of the report, one of the
anchors asked Mr. Wilson whether, or not there were any pharmacies that did not
adhere to this practice, and he said that Costco consistently charged little over their cost
for the generic drugs.
I went to the Costco site, where you can look up any drug, and get its online price. It
says that the in-store prices are consistent with the online prices. I was appalled. Just to
give you one example from my own experience, I had to use the drug, Compazine,
which helps prevent nausea in chemo patients. I used the generic equivalent, which
cost $54.99 for 60 pills at CVS. I checked the price at Costco, and I could have bought

100 pills for $19.89. For 145 of my pain pills, I paid $72.57.
I could have got 150 at
Costco for $28.08.

I would like to mention, that although Costco is a
'membership' type store, you do NOT
have to be a member to buy prescriptions there, as it is a
federally regulated substance.
You just tell them at the door that you wish to use the
pharmacy, and they will let you in.
This is true in Canada, too. I went there this past Thursday
and asked them.
I am asking each of you to please help me by copying this
letter, and passing it into your
own e-mail, and send it to everyone you know with an e-
mail address. Enough already!

If you are willing to accept the fact that treating allergies with drugs only prolongs the inevitable, and that doctors don't always have the right answer, and that there are other ways to overcome allergies without drugs, then this eBook will be able to find the right answer for you. It will explain how the body works so that you can understand what you are taking, and why you are taking it. If you just want to know what you need to add to your diet, then jump to the SUMMARY CHAPTER at the end of this eBook and start a short shopping list.

There is no one size fits all for allergy sufferers as each person has their own set of unique dietary needs. As if that wasn't enough of a challenge, these needs will also change over time. So, what worked in your 20's might not necessarily work in your 40's. For this reason it is important to understand how the body works so that you can

give it what it needs during these times of growth
and stress. Eventually, you will be able to read your
body like a book and respond to it accordingly no
matter what age you are, and no matter where the
allergy seems to come from.

Common Treatments

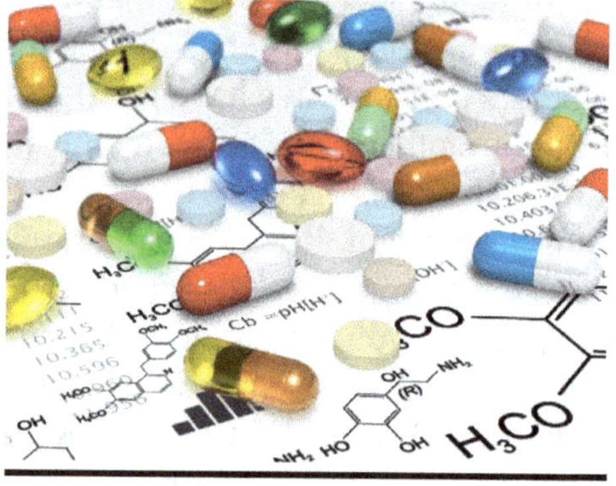

There are so many kinds of allergy treatments
available these days that it can leave the allergy
sufferer thinking that he only needs to find the right
one for him, and then his world will return to
normal. The problem is that none of these drug
related treatments will actually cure allergies; they
only manipulate the symptoms, and provide a

temporary relief. Eventually, the side effects will manifest, and the patient will have to move on to something else, or start an additional drug related treatment for the side effects of their allergy medicine. All of the leading allergy treatments come with extensive warnings and side effects, but to someone who is suffering, anything is better than a pounding headache, sneezing, stuffy nose and all the miserable feelings that allergies bring.
Among the most common treatments are;

- Anti-histamines
- Decongestants
- Steroids
- Bronchodilators
- Mast cell stabilizers
- Leukotriene Modifiers, and
- Immunotherapy (allergy shots)

Allergy shots are thought to be the most effective form of therapy because they help the body develop a resistance to the allergen over time, but this only works if the individuals' body is healthy and has the nutrition it needs to build up and maintain a defense. Unless the patient is taking steps to improve his overall health, allergy shots are similar to whipping a dead horse; they are forcing the body to do what it would do on its own when it is working properly in the first place.

History

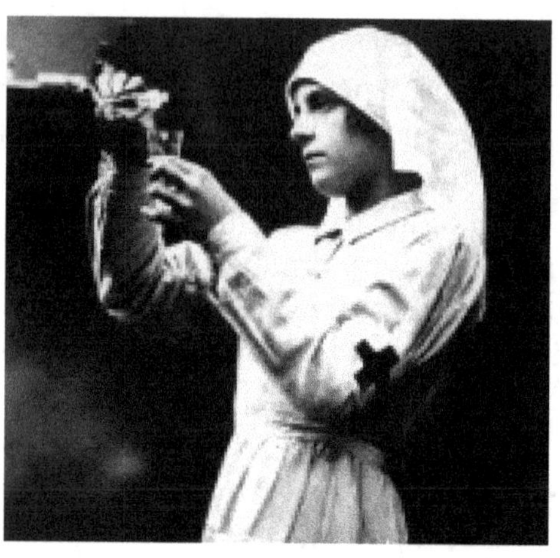

Specific immunotherapy has been practiced for almost 100 years and recorded as early as 1900. By 1911, physicians Noon and Freeman[5] were practicing immunotherapy by injection with great results. There was a significant rise in research to treat allergies in the 1920's and 1930's when the focus became simply finding the right dose and method of introduction. For pollen, mold, dust mites, stinging insects, cat, and dog allergies, the allergen injection method was the standard, until doctors started to gradually abandon this therapy after several food allergy fatalities occurred.

Sublingual immunotherapy was again revived in 1969 predominantly by David Morris[6]. Even though this method of treating allergies is still in use today, treating food allergies seems to be a delicate matter and is therefore still being researched on a case by case basis. Once again, this is because each person has their own unique needs concerning allergic reactions. The idea here is to build up the body's defense system so that it will fight any allergen no matter where it comes from. In my opinion, gradually introducing allergens to a compromised immune system is risky at best.

Immunotherapy was again revived for inhalant allergens back in the 1970's[7], and while greatly improved, finding the right dose and the best way to introduce the allergen varies greatly. After almost a century of testing and trials, there is still no standard in place where external methods of immunotherapy is applied. *However, building up the adrenal glands, and the liver will change this situation for anyone who is serious about resolving their allergies once and for all.*

This is easy to understand, as there is no magic bullet that will solve the allergy sufferer's problems, and there never will be; because every person's needs vary greatly according the levels of stress, and these needs fluctuate throughout the year. The focus should be on improving the individuals' overall health, rather than trying to find the 'perfect' marketable product that will target just the reaction.

In the end, the majority of the medical industry is looking at their patients from the wrong side of the fence. Instead of introducing another external substance that will solve the internal problems, a good healer will look at how to get the body to the place where it can heal itself from the inside out.

It is funny to me to watch the allergy commercials woven throughout our American society. They will spend 30 seconds telling us how wonderful their product is, and then follow up with 90 seconds of all the horrible things that will happen to you if you continue to take it. They will get an extremely fast talker to run down the side effects as if they were nothing at all, and simply something that their 'legal department' requires them to share…If you can't see the irony in that then you are taking way too many allergy meds.

Side Effects

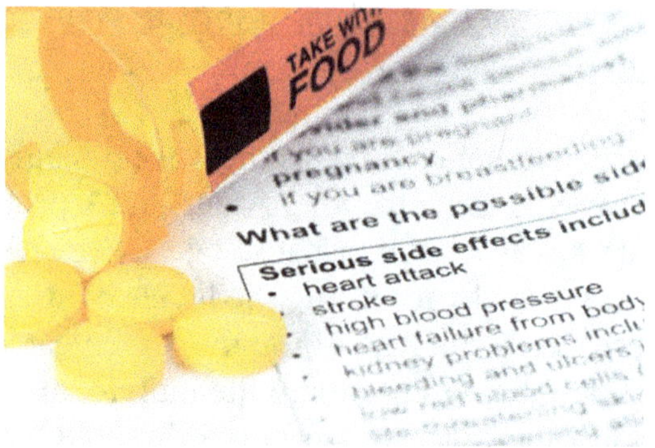

Some of these side effects that are thrown at us so nonchalantly include;
- Drowsiness from antihistamines
- High blood pressure
- Insomnia
- Irritability and
- Restricted urination from decongestants

- Steroids have numerous potential side effects of their own, including:
  - ➤ Weight gain
  - ➤ Fluid retention
  - ➤ High blood pressure
  - ➤ Growth suppression
  - ➤ Diabetes
  - ➤ Cataracts
  - ➤ Osteoporosis
  - ➤ Muscle weakness
  - ➤ Coughs
  - ➤ Hoarseness, and
  - ➤ Yeast infections

Natural remedies rarely get this much media attention because they have no side effects. So when the patients' allergies disappear, the patient will assume that they just grew out of them; or it was a mystery on how that happened. 'Oh well, no allergies today, it was a good day, don't know why…'

There is no drama attached to Natural Healing; subsequently, they get no publicity at all. Many people assume that they can't be that good if there are no side effects. The ridiculous notion that allergy treatments without side effects are not capable of treating severe allergies is so pervasive partly because allergies are so miserable, there must be a price to pay in order to get rid of them.

Imagine all your symptoms simply fading away with no fanfare at all. This happens all the time, but most people act like it was just a 'good day' that

they will never understand. The truth is, building up the body's adrenal glands and feeding it nutritionally rich foods/ supplements during times of stress will restore its ability to fight against allergens without the aid of synthetic drugs.
If certain minimum vitamin requirements are maintained, the body will over time grow stronger; stay allergy free AND be healthier on several fronts, not just when it comes to allergies.

One very common example comes from Grandma's salt solutions. We were told to just gargle with salt water, or eat some hot, salty, chicken soup. In these modern times, these solutions are thought to be too old fashioned; and can't possibly work in this day and age, and yet, many of the leading OTC (over the counter) drugs list sodium as their number one ingredient. They continue to sell simple salt solutions for $3 to $5 a box, surrounded by a flashy advertising campaign, when all the while a bottle of Gatorade and a small bag of chips will do the same thing for a lot less. The reason is simple. Eating salt will raise the blood sodium levels, and therefore pull water out of the tissues, drying up watery eyes and a running nose.
Yes, it is that simple.

While salt is certainly not a cure all for allergies, it is one simple method that does work to some degree. For those on a low salt diet, there are other ways to help reduce swelling that we will address later on. For now it is enough to understand that if you are serious about improving your health, then

you are going to have to make the decision to feed
your body what it needs, and not necessarily just
what you feel like eating because it tastes good.

Nutritional-Therapy also addresses these issues in
other publications[8]. There are several things that
affect the chronic allergy sufferer and only by
treating the entire person will they be able to
overcome these issues once and for all.

What Are Allergies?

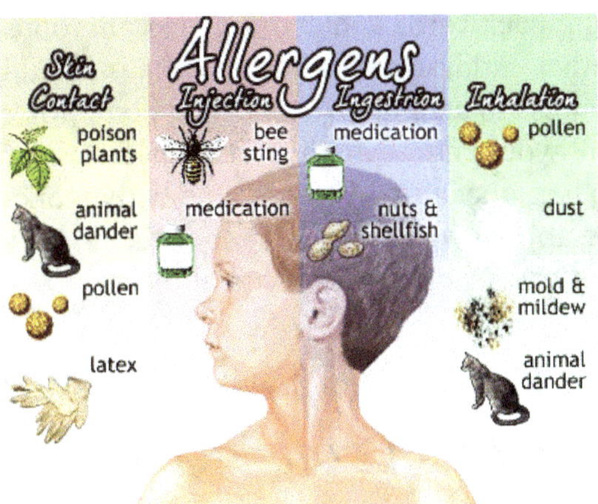

Allergies are the many different ways the human
body reacts to allergens when they enter the blood.
These allergens are more often than not nothing
more than very small protein particles that can enter
through the skin, mucous membranes, respiratory

and intestinal tract. They usually enter the body without us even knowing it through some routine, daily activity. This is why trying to limit contact with an allergen in order to avoid an allergic reaction is not really a practical way to deal with them. They are everywhere, and more often than not we are not even aware that we are in contact with allergens until we have a reaction to it. So it's easy to see that trying to limit foods for fear of an allergic reaction is not the best way to deal with the signs and symptoms. This only depletes the body of much needed nutrition at the exact time that the person needs it most. This is why the focus should be on building up a strong body so it can fight allergens the way it was designed to, instead of stepping backwards and avoiding certain foods altogether. Adding drugs into the mix only adds more stress to an already weakened condition. While I would not dismiss allergy medications altogether, once you learn how the body works, you will be able to wean yourself off of them gradually without triggering a possibly fatal reaction.

Never stop allergy medication without your doctor's approval.

Some allergies, particularly respiratory allergies can be fatal. Improving the diet will allow you to gradually step away from the medications simply because you will not be experiencing any symptoms that require them.

Allergies are well known to be 'stress diseases', because they seem to flare up when people are under a disproportionate amount of stress. While people don't always recognize them as allergies, some of the most common allergies people suffer from are;

- Rashes
- Eczema
- Hives
- Hay fever
- Asthma
- Headaches
- Runny or stuffy nose
- Sinus infections, and
- Digestive-problems

Interestingly enough, there are separate and specific drugs sold for each one of these symptoms, raking in billions of dollars every year. However, in reality they all stem from the same fundamental problem; the bodies inability to rid itself of a foreign allergen.

<u>Vaccines</u>

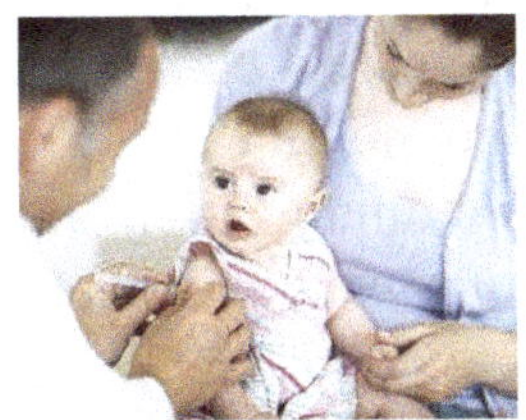

Getting a vaccine is a common way to discover allergies. Vaccines are a small amount of some foreign substance injected into the blood that will give the immune system an introduction to it. By introducing a small part of a foreign substance to the immune system, this will allow the body to develop white blood cells that will attack it if that allergen ever shows up again on a larger scale. Immunizations basically give the body a chance to recognize a foreign substance, so that it won't be taken by surprise by it in the future.

Recent studies concerning vaccines are showing that infants and children are simply not ready to be assaulted at such a young age with a dose of vaccines, yet they are required before kids are allowed to go to school. Parents should think long and hard before allowing their kids to be vaccinated at such a young age.[9]

So we need to ask ourselves, why do some people have violent reactions to foreign substances, while others never notice them? Simply put, because some people's immune systems are better able to rally a defense than others. A healthy immune system is not something we are either born with, or we aren't. They are created and nurtured by giving the body specific nutrition. There are a few specific vitamins that will charge the immune system so that it will be ready to attack an immunization and prevent the foreign body from causing any damage once inside.

 If you are one of those people that just can't eat vegetable, then at least take a B-vitamin supplement along with some Vitamin C. This will give your body something to work with and get you started on the right road to recovery.

FYI ~ The Caduceus

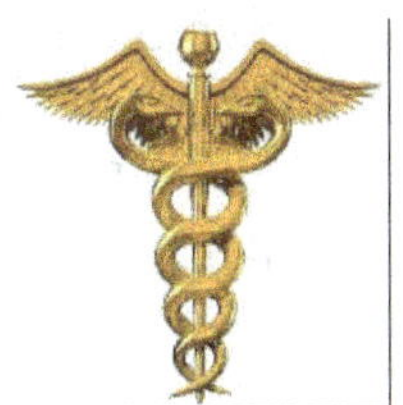

I am not saying do away with vaccinations, what I am saying give your body the B-Vitamins, Vitamin C and Protein it needs to rally a strong defense. The caduceus is a good example of why vaccinations do work and why we should not dismiss them altogether. Man was made from this earth, and from the earth we can find our cures. This is a good example of how vaccinations work. The Caduceus is the worldwide symbol that represents the practice of medicine, signified by 2 snakes wrapped around a cross. Originally found in the Bible, Numbers 21:4-9, when Moses wrapped bronze snakes around a cross as a sign that would protect the people of Israel against fiery serpents. It also represents how in order to treat the venom from a snake bite, a doctor needs to inject the anti-venom to counter act it. Thus, from the source of illness is found the cure. The same is true today; vaccinations introduce a small amount of allergen to the body in order to give the immune system a small, weakened exposure. This way the body will have time to develop white blood cells that will attack the allergen in case it shows up again in the future. By feeding the body what it needs to fight infection, it will be ready to combat an allergen in the same way. So, while we are immunizing our children, make sure we are also giving them enough nutrition to be able to fight the allergen once it is injected. It doesn't take much, a multi-vitamin, vitamin water, a protein shake. Adding these simple things to the diet will have a tremendous impact on your child's overall health.

<u>Why Me?</u>

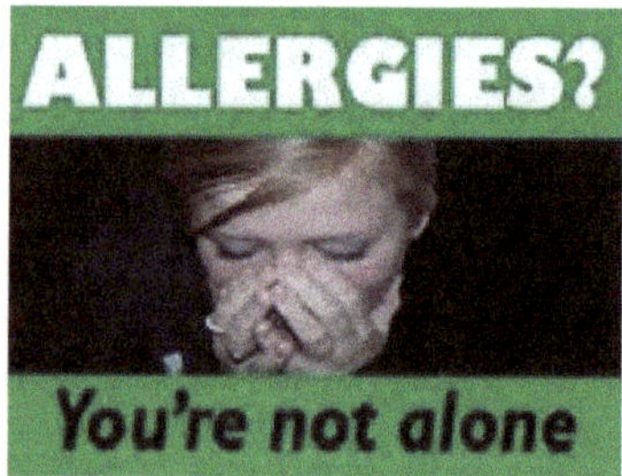

People who suffer from allergies will often wonder 'Why do I have them, and everyone else around me can endure this type of environment?' Doctors will often say; 'you just can't tolerate that… this is your specific problem…you need to learn how to live with it because there is no cure for allergies.'

In Truth; this is rarely the case. More often than not, allergies can be treated not by avoiding the allergen, but by building up good health, and equipping the body to handle an allergen once it enters the body. So instead of avoiding a small grocery store of healthy foods on the chance that something won't agree with the individual, treatment should focus on building up their liver and adrenal glands to the point that they are producing their own cortisone and other anti-allergy chemicals. Even adding nothing more than vitamins will make a big improvement until the individual learns to eat in a manner that will restore health instead of just bogging it down.

It is far easier to process allergens out of the body than it is to run away from them; they are in the food we eat, the water we drink, and the air we breathe. As stated before, avoiding certain foods will make matters worse because it will rob the body of desperately needed nutrition required to rebuild the body during these exact times of stress in adults, and rapid growth in children.

The Cost

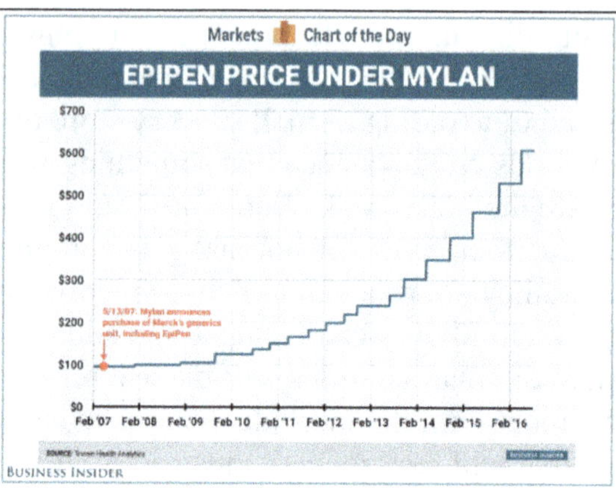

Many are those who say "vitamins are too expensive…" and yet they will hand over thousands of dollars each year for prescription meds that only aggravate, and compound their problems.

People claim that they can't afford to take a day off work, and then continue to work through the weekend. They will push their body to the point that they get admitted to a hospital, but still refuse to alter their lifestyle in order to prevent stress from building up to the breaking point time and time again.

People will seek a doctor's advice about how to restore their fading health, only to reject his advice, and continue to eat and act like they always have; taking a chance that they might somehow get a different result this time.

Guess what- none of that works.

All metabolic[10] diseases respond to diet and nutrition, and can be improved by improving the diet. The biggest failure found in alternative medicine is not the results, but the people's inability to discipline themselves enough to eat what their body needs. Unfortunately, most people have collectively grown comfortable with letting someone else take care of us, so we have lost control- and responsibility- for our own general health. In America, people are so conditioned to eat only what tastes good that many refuse to even put a vegetable on their plate, much less eat one. It is somewhat understandable in children, but adults deal with far more stress, and have more issues with aging, and therefore need to alter their diet as they get older to one that is more nutrient rich, and one that will restore and maintain their good health. The human body must ingest the nutrients found in fruits, vegetables, meats, fish and dairy if it is going to function right. If a body can't tolerate these foods, that person should at least take supplements that will provide what their body needs in order to continue to perform without failing. Vitamins and minerals are a lot less costly than prescription drugs, in more ways than one.

It's In the Family...

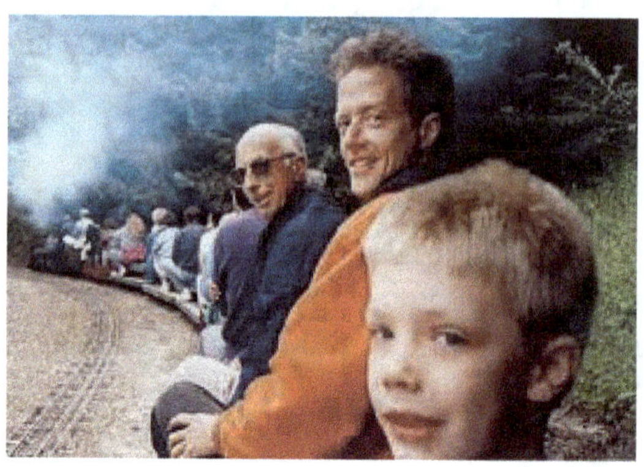

Allergy studies have been going on for decades.
When the adrenal glands of test animals are taken
out to simulate adrenal exhaustion, this will prevent
cortisone from reaching the blood[11]. Without this
vital relationship allergen injections are always
severe, and sometimes fatal[12]. Yet, the same
injections into healthy animals will have no reaction
at all. Both in animals and humans, injections of
cortisone will alleviate allergic reactions, but only
temporarily.

Allergy sufferers are notorious for living lifestyles
that include eating diets that are high carbohydrates;
low in protein, living with insufficient sleep,
emotional ups and downs, infections, and side
effects from other synthetic drugs. The allergen is
little more than the straw that broke the camel's
back[13].

Stress increases the bodies need for all nutrients, so
when a victim of allergies starts to limit foods that
they think are causing allergies, they are really just

adding to the problem. It is exactly at times like this that the body needs all the nutrition it can get. Adding protein shakes and vitamins is a safe and effective way to supplement the body, while gradually introducing healthy foods back into the diet as the body grows stronger.

For example, children with hives, asthma, or eczema improve greatly when only liver tablets; and/or a B- complex vitamin supplement were given them[14]. This one change alone will alter the lives of thousands of people.

Certain people are genetically predisposed to high requirements of certain nutrients, based on their family history. Once these are discovered, and added back into the diet in an appropriate amount, tests show that allergies will almost always disappear within a few weeks, and often stay away forever[15]. This is also why so many kids outgrow their allergies, because as they get older, they will typically eat a broader, more varied diet, and eventually supply the missing nutrients they weren't getting as a kid.

Bread and the B Vitamins

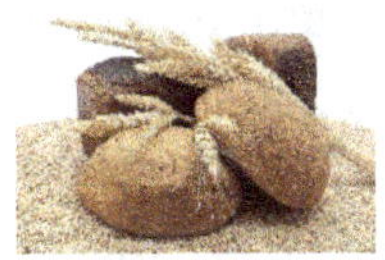

After WWII, the FDA found themselves is the middle of several trade wars that decided the fate of many food manufacturers. With the increased production of mass marketed processed foods, manufacturers were looking for ways to extend the shelf life of their products, and therefore increasing their presence in the marketplace. The end result was that manufacturers ended up stripping almost everything of nutritional value out of their foods, leaving only the remnants of what the food once was. The biggest impact was in our daily bread. Producers were stripping the wheat germ off the wheat, and making bread with only the white, starchy flour, leaving the end product nutritionally void.

After seeing a sudden rise in reoccurring health issues across the United States, particularly beriberi[16] and pellagra[17], the government stepped in and declared that "…Recipe standards for enriched foods helped eliminate a number of nutritional deficiency diseases [beriberi and pellagra] in the post-war era, particularly in southern states…"[18], and thus emerged 'white bread- with 8 essential vitamins and minerals!'[19]
It was only 'enriched' with about 1/10th of its original nutritional value, but because it was added back into the flour, enriched was the term the regulators chose to use. This one simple alteration to the American diet alone, is accountable for countless health issues that many people still suffer to this day[20]. Without the nutrients and oils found in freshly ground whole grain that includes the wheat germ, bread is little more than a sponge that will simply fill the stomach to keep it quiet. When kids

with asthma, hives, and eczema started taking higher doses of vitamin B12, one of the main ingredients found in wheat germ, their symptoms improved greatly with just the addition of this one simple vitamin.[21] One quick way to change this fact is by adding a tablespoon of wheat germ back into all bread products. It has no taste, but brings a handful of nutrition without your kids knowing it. Every time you make a sandwich, or eat pasta just sprinkle a tablespoon of wheat germ on the meal, and you will find your child's health improving exponentially in a matter of days.

It must be said however, that the B vitamins are water soluble, so they are not stored anywhere in the body. This means that they need to be eaten every day in order to maintain good health. They should also be taken all together in the form of a B-complex vitamin in order to avoid any imbalances. Because they are water soluble, it is hard, if not impossible, to take too many since any excess will simply be excreted out of the body. However, when imbalances occur, they can make a person feel a little nauseous. This is why it is a good idea to take them in the form of wheat germ, or with a little food and water. Vitamin Water adds a little flavor to ordinary water, and supplies more than enough of the required daily doses of all the B vitamins. Because these vitamins are mixed in the water, the chances of getting that nauseous feeling are remote and something not known to happen.

If vitamin water is not available near you, you can purchase wheat germ at almost any local grocery store. This is the part of the grain that is stripped away, and contains all the nutrition. Simply sprinkling a tablespoon of wheat germ on cereal, bread, pizza dough, anywhere you are eating bread products, you will be adding back 23 nutrients, and more protein per ounce than can be found in most meat products.[22]

Supplements

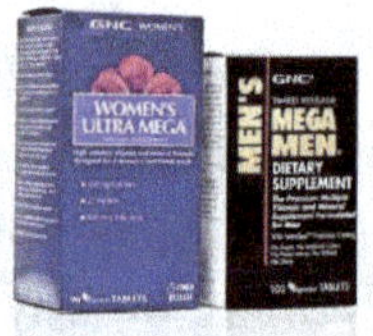

One of the more popular studies held at the Antibiotic Medical Clinic back in the 1950's found that

> '...32 allergic children [who] suffered from bronchial asthma, and allergic eczema were given;
> generous amounts of protein,
> no refined carbohydrates,
> adequate essential fatty acids,
> daily doses of 600 mg of Vitamin C,
> 32 mg of vitamin E,
> 20,000 units of vitamin A,
> 800 units of vitamin D and a moderate supply of the B vitamins, most recovered within a month, and all within 2 months'[23]

Although this sounds like a lot to add back into the diet, in today's health conscience society, all of these nutrients can be eaten in one meal and serve the body throughout the day. There isn't one missing ingredient that we can take to safeguard against allergic reactions, but it is rather a diet that is high in protein, low in carbohydrates, includes fresh fruits and vegetables, and plenty of water. In light of how our foods are processed in today's modern American diet, supplements are more likely to supply what we need; as we can hardly eat enough processed food to get the required nutrition. Unless the food you eat is obtained before it was processed, and you cook it yourself, chances are they have already lost much of their nutritional value by the time it reaches our plates.[24]

Good Digestion and the Auto Immune Disease

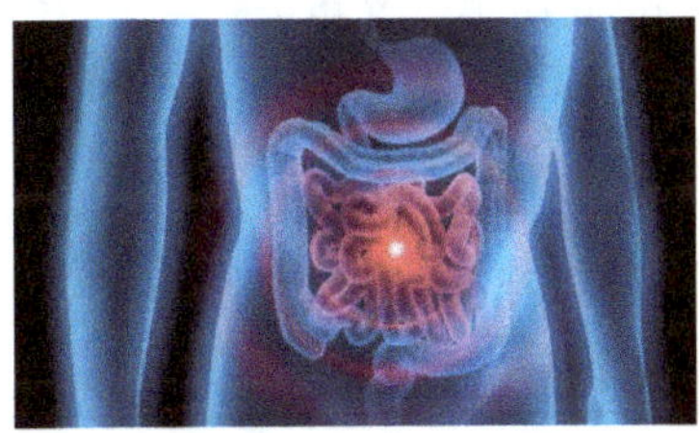

Food allergies most often occur because food is not completely digested. This partially digested food can get into the blood stream, become an irritant, and then cause any number of allergic reactions. When protein is not completely digested, the amino acid 'histidine' is changed by decomposing intestinal bacteria into the annoying 'histamine'[25].

 Histamines are found in higher than average amounts in the blood of people with allergies.[26] By blocking histamines with 'anti-histamine' drugs a person will be able to effectively stop the allergic reaction, and have temporary relief from all the miseries of allergies. However, the key word here is 'temporary'.

Instead of taking more drugs, a healthy liver will produce the enzyme 'histaminase', which quickly oxidizes any histamine that the body produces, enabling the body to intercept this chain reaction before a full-blown allergy occurs[27].

When the body is under stress, it can also break down tissue protein[28], another process known to produce histamine. This is why some people can actually have allergic reactions to things like the sun, extreme heat or bitter cold.[29] These conditions can be so physically stressful to some people that they will actually trigger a reaction that will break down the tissue protein of their body in order to use the proteins for the bodies' self-defense.

This is something that many people simply don't understand, and modern medicine has labeled an 'Auto-Immune' disease. The majority of people walking around in society will hear of someone claiming to be allergic to the sun, heat or cold, and immediately consider these claims absurd, or made just to get attention.

In Truth, these seemingly everyday occurrences can cause some undernourished people enough physical stress that their body will automatically begin to start this allergic reaction of turning on their own body. This process of breaking down tissue protein will in turn produce histamine and cause an allergic reaction. It is not a sign of emotional instability, or a case of the body turning on itself, but a simple physical reaction from an undernourished body trying to acquire enough protein to keep the engines running. This person is just trying to adjust to a sudden and sharp change in the environment. By adding protein to the diet, this will do more for the auto-immune patient than any number of drugs they can take to silence the symptoms.

The Role of the Liver

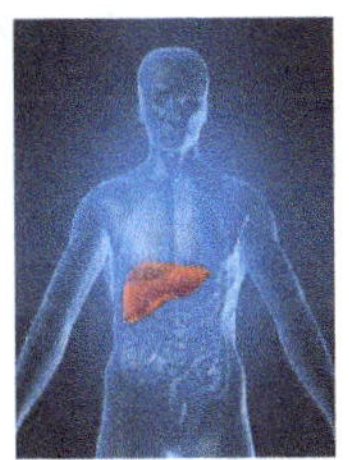

As mentioned before, a healthy liver will produce the enzyme 'histaminase', which will oxidize any histamine that the body produces[30] no matter where it came from. However, the liver of people that are stressed or eating a poor diet are unable to produce enough histaminase to combat growing levels of histamine once an allergic reaction starts.

The condition of the liver is one reason why over the counter anti-histamines can be considered so harmful. Synthetically produced anti-histamines tend to damage the liver over time, so much so that they will cause the liver to stop producing histaminase altogether and leave the poor person chemically dependent of the store-bought version[31].

These research results were taken from studies that considered anti-histamine use a success.[32] The prevailing medical thought is to stop the allergies; not treat the patient. As far as research is considered, OTC antihistamines are a success, despite the fact that they continually damage the very organ that was designed to treat allergies naturally in the first place.

Thank God the liver is an organ that can regenerate itself. When given the right diet, the liver can correct itself, and repair the negative effects of this very common long term drug use.

"The human liver is one of the few organs in the body that

can regenerate from as little as 25 percent of its tissue,"

-Seth Karp, assistant professor of surgery at Harvard Medical School, Boston.[33]

Once the diet and the liver have been restored, the liver will be able to produce enough histaminase to automatically stop allergic reactions from ever getting started in the first place.

The Role of the Adrenal Glands

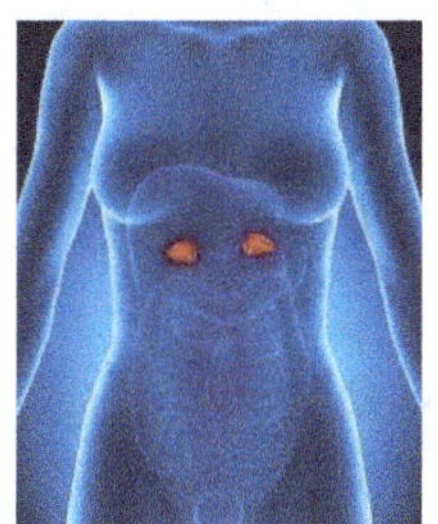

One of the more common forms of relief for allergies is a shot of cortisone. Since this is more effective given as a shot directly into the affected area, shots are taken from the hand of any licensed professional. While it is effective, it requires trips to the doctor's office, waiting in line, and is generally a major intrusion into the lives of those who need them.

Since the adrenal glands can naturally produce cortisone by themselves when they are healthy, it makes good sense to get the adrenals working rather than running to the doctor every time someone starts to tear and sneeze. This is no easy fix though. It takes a well-supplied diet high in protein and all the vitamins and minerals to get the adrenals in top condition, but in today's health conscience society meeting these demands has never been easier.

Vitamin B5, Also Known As Pantothenic Acid

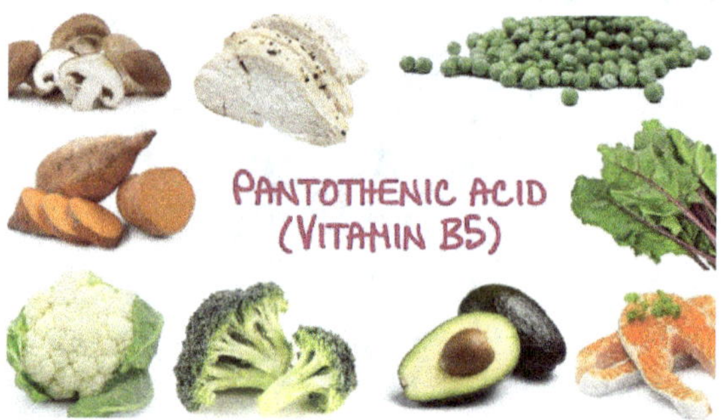

Vitamin B5 is also known as Pantothenic acid, a water-soluble vitamin that as said before; cannot be stored in the body so it needs to be eaten every day. Vitamin B5 is listed in the ingredients of many foods as 'Pantothenic acid'. You should be aware of this if you are reading labels. Why is this name change done? I don't know. It seems that it would be much simpler to keep the B's in order; numbered 1,2,3,5,6,7,9 &12.

Vitamin B5 is most commonly found in fresh fruits and vegetables and inside the husks of grain. It is also one of the main ingredients manufacturers strip from foods in order to get a longer shelf life. If you are the typical American then you are no doubt eating far too few fruits and vegetables, despite the fact that we have them at our disposal 24-hours a day; 7 days a week in virtually every corner market. Sorry mom, 'fruit flavored snacks' and 'lots of orange juice' doesn't count.

Everyone needs to eat real fruit. The pasteurization of commercial foods destroys much of their nutritional value,[34] and there are still other nutrients found in real food that we haven't even discovered yet. They all need to work together to provide optimum health.

For many animals, Vitamin B5/Pantothenic Acid is a mandatory nutrient. They need it to synthesize coenzyme-A (CoA) as well as to synthesize and metabolize proteins, carbohydrates, and fats.[35] Some animals are found to need 20 times the average amount of B5/Pantothenic acid because of their genetic makeup.[36] The same can be said of humans. There are certain families that require far more of this vitamin than the general populace and without it, they suffer far more than the rest of us do, too.[37] With the average intake being somewhere around 4-5 mg daily, there are some families that need as much as 200 mg a day to maintain good health.[38] Since it is water soluble there is no need to be concerned about getting too much, any excess is simply lost in the urine. Drinking plenty of Vitamin Water is a great way to remedy this shortage.

Since cortisone also cannot be produced without Vitamin B5 (Pantothenic Acid)[39], it makes sense to add this to the diet as one of the first supplements. Symptoms of Vitamin B5/Pantothenic acid deficiencies are very similar to those of allergies;

Fatigue
Listlessness
Poor appetite
Digestive problems
Headache
Irritability
Nervousness
Depression

Quarreling
The need to sleep
Recent respiratory infections, and a
Large number of 'eosinophils' cells in the blood and lymph... just to name a few.[40]

The addition of Pantothenic acid alone has been known to effect allergies more than any other nutrient[41], and when combined with the cortisone produced from the adrenal glands, it is a very powerful defense against all allergens, no matter where they come from, or how severe the onslaught.

Vitamin C- Dedicated to Linus Pauling

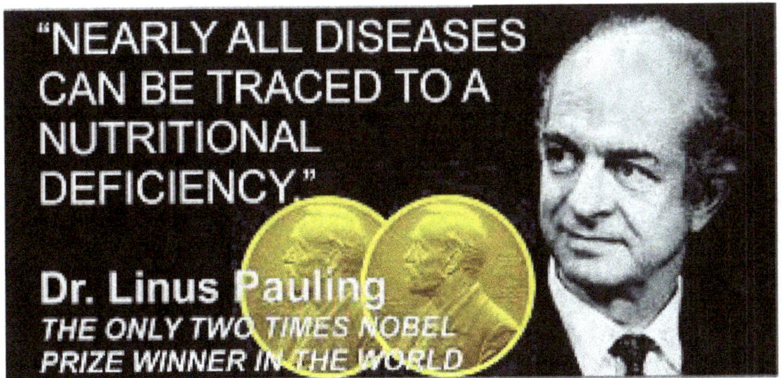

Vitamin C plays a very large role in getting the adrenals to produce more cortisone. It is always found to be in very low levels within the blood of persons suffering from allergies.[42] Vitamin C also increases both the production of, and the effectiveness of cortisone produced by the adrenal cortex.[43]

Vitamin C, Vitamin B5/ Pantothenic acid, and Vitamin B6 each have their own anti-histamine effects on the body,[44] but when combined they will decrease the amount of certain undesired red blood cells called 'eosinophils',[45] and help prevent them from increasing in the blood.[46] Since eosinophilis are found at high levels in the blood of people who suffer from allergies[47] it makes sense to address them at this time, too.

In both animals and humans, the amount of vitamin C found in the blood of allergic persons is considered very low as compared to their peers.[48] Vitamin C is so important to so many functions within the body, I am sure that it is only a matter of time before Nutritional-Therapy will produce an eBook on just this vitamin alone. Linus Pauling[49] laid the foundation for vitamin C back in the 1950's and 1960's with his many works in this field and his findings deserve to be expounded on even to this day. While he was ridiculed and criticized for his 'theories-eventually proven facts' -about vitamin C, he went on to be the only recipient of two individual Nobel Prizes[50] in Biochemistry and another one for Peace. His work is well respected and highly referenced even to this day. His theories have now been accepted and proven true over and over again, and he stands out as one of the most accomplished and successful philanthropists of our time. Learning more about his work, and all the benefits of vitamin C is something that those interested would really benefit from.

One of the other most promising effects of Vitamin C is that it is instrumental in detoxifying the body of all toxins, as well as allergens.[51] However, vitamin C is used up in this process at a rate proportional to the amount of toxins absorbed.[52] This means that if you are exposed to cigarette smoke, are eating foods with pesticides, or breathing unclean & stale air, you would naturally need more Vitamin C than someone who is not subjected to this kind of environment. Because of this detoxifying effect, sudden, large amounts of Vitamin C supplements have been known to cause rashes and diarrhea in some people as the body begins to rid itself of various substances.

When Vitamin C reduces swelling in the intestines and bowels, they start to release all the bile that was trapped in the folds. This is also the cause of a temporary bout with diarrhea that some people experience while adding this to their diet. If this is the case with you simply stop taking so much Vitamin C and start eating natural sources such as fresh fruits and vegetables. After these negative effects subside, you can start adding smaller doses of Vitamin C until your balance is found. 250 mg-500 gm a day is a good starting point.

This detoxifying and anti-histamine effect of vitamin C has long been known by the medical community,[53] but with the easy access of over the counter drugs, and cortisone shots, the public switched their focus; and responsibility off themselves and on to the quick fix that the pharmaceutical industry has to offer.

Drug Addiction Isn't Always Illegal

In the natural, humans, moneys and guinea pigs are the only mammals that don't make their own Vitamin C. All the others that do, make it consistently at about 35 mg for every pound that they weigh. A typical vitamin C therapy would consist of approximately 300 mg every 15 minutes for a visible improvement within the hour,[54] but this was not fast enough for 'modern man'. He wanted to inhale something and get immediate relief within minutes or even seconds in many cases, and think about it later. There are times when that is appropriate, particularly in acute situations, but for the average allergy sufferer this is not the answer.

The problem with pharmaceuticals is that people forgot all about natural therapy and quickly became dependent on synthetic drugs. Eventually, everyone including the medical community forgot about vitamin C altogether, and the people became addicted to their puffer. A simple 1500 to 2000 mg daily would go a long way to prevent allergy attacks,[55] and prime the body to be ready for any allergen that decided to cross its path anytime in the future.

Today's timed release tablets [chelated] make it possible to take one vitamin C supplement in the morning, and have it slowly release vitamin C all through the day. There are also several good soft chew sources of vitamin C that can be eaten like candy. With all the varieties of vitamin C available in the market there is no excuse for anyone to not get enough in this day and age.

In addition to assisting the adrenal glands in producing more cortisone, Vitamin C makes this cortisone more effective in the process.[56] Vitamin C also decreases the permeability of cells[57], and has an anti-histamine action all its own, that is beyond the scope of this writing.

<u>Cell Permeability</u>

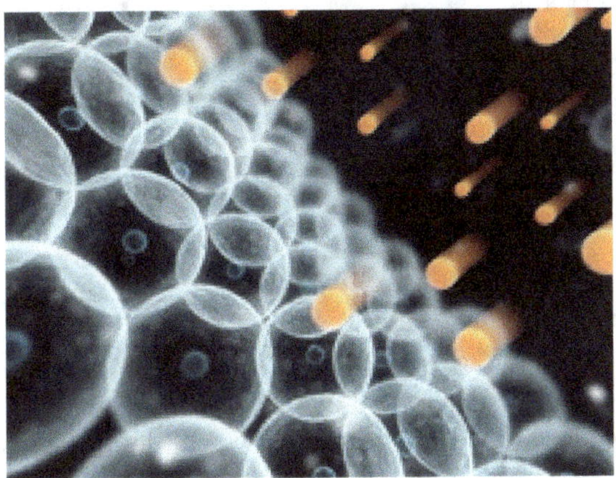

In summary, the following chapter refers to the various nutrients that are needed to start combatting allergies by increasing cell permeability. If you cannot find a way to incorporate them into your diet- then take supplements. One good, high quality multi-vitamin and a protein shake daily should be enough to put you back in balance. If you want more, the following chapters will spell is out for you as well.

<u>Vitamin C</u>

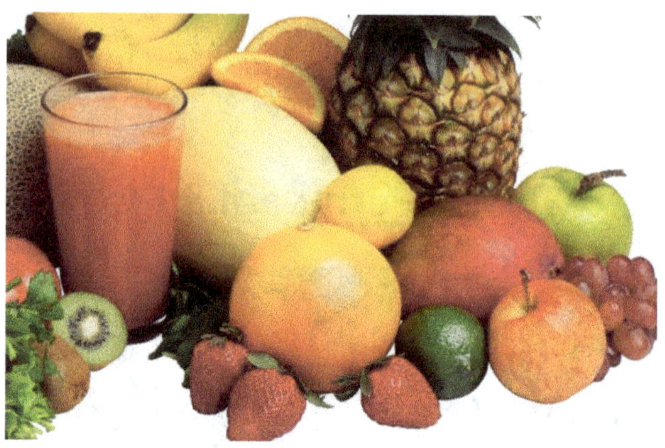

Another function of Vitamin C is the increased production of collagen.[58] Collagen is the glue that helps to hold cells together.[59] When collagen levels are low, cell structure is weakened, and permeability is high, allowing valuable nutrients to leak out and annoying allergens to seep in.

Without generous amounts of naturally produced collagen, the cells can easily break down and become more fragile, as well as permeable. This explains why people who don't have enough vitamin C bruise more easily, have more nosebleeds, and experience bleeding gums.[60] Without enough collagen to hold the cells together, they begin to break down and will rupture from even the slightest bump. A simple knock on the arm to a healthy person will produce nothing, but if the cell stability is weak that same bump will rupture the cells, and cause blood to leak out, causing the familiar bruising that we can all see.

Protein

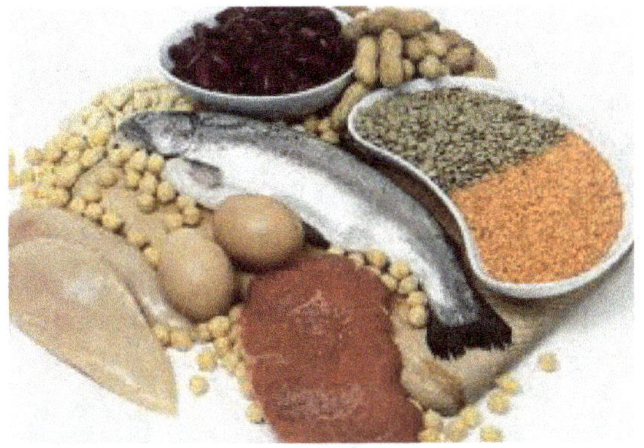

Having a decent protein intake is also important as stress can often happen very quickly, causing the body to break down protein in the tissues if no other source is available. Another case of the mislabeled "Auto-Immune" disease. The body will only turn on itself if the diet doesn't provide what it needs to function. The 'Auto-Immune Disease' is not a disease at all, but an allergy that only needs to be addressed with the right nutritional balance.

Not only does this breakdown of tissue protein increase the production of histamine; it will eventually take its toll on all the tissues of the body and interfere with other daily, vital functions. A minimum intake of protein should be 80 grams a day for men and 60 grams a day for women. More won't hurt, but this should be the minimum. If you are active or larger than most other people you can certainly take more. Actually, since protein burns carbohydrates in the digestion process, eating a high protein diet will actually help you burn fat and keep your energy levels high as well. The only risk in high protein diets is that they tend to be higher in saturated fats and cholesterols. However, it you add 21 grains of lecithin to the meal, it will balance these fats out so that won't be a problem.[61] Nutritional-Therapy has a separate eBook on this subject, which can be found on Amazon if you would like to know more. You can also contact us on our web site www.Nutritional-Therapy.us

<u>Essential Fatty Acids and Vitamin E</u>

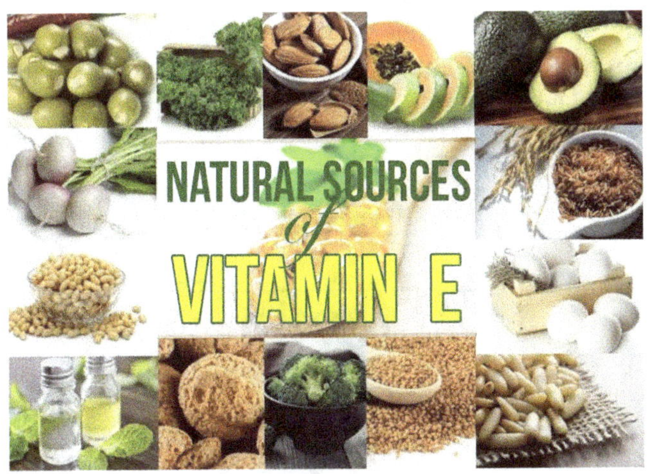

According to Wikipedia;
Essential fatty acids, or EFAs, are fatty acids that humans and other animals must ingest because the body requires them for good health but cannot synthesize them. The term "essential fatty acid" refers to fatty acids required for biological processes, and not those that only act as fuel.[62]

These acids are linolenic acid, arachidonic acid and linolenic acid. If these are lacking from the diet or damaged by a lack of oxygen, this will also contribute to cell permeability. One way to increase the beneficial effects of oxygen is to supplement with Vitamin E. Because breast milk is very rich in vitamin E, infants that are fed breast milk rarely have allergies, but formula fed babies seem to experience them ten-fold[63]. Vitamin E reduces the cells need for oxygen and therefore preserves them from oxidation.[64] This way, cells can use oxygen without being harmed by it; and these essential oils will have greater ability to do all the things that they were designed to do once inside the body.

<u>Vitamin A</u>

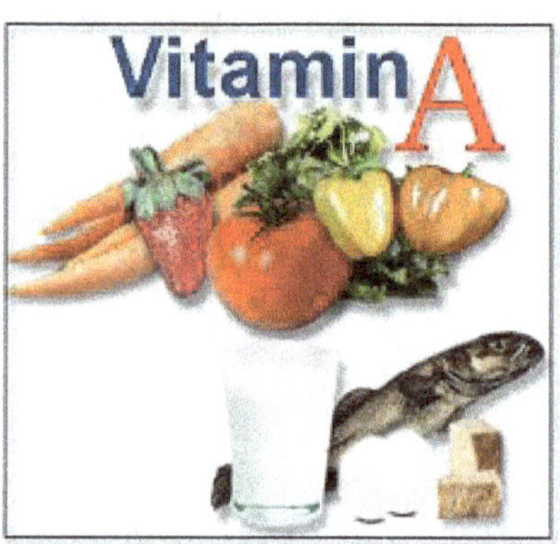

Vitamin A also plays a role in cell permeability by building up the many layers of skin, and the mucous linings in the nose and stomach.[65] Vitamin A is another one of those supplements that brings improved health in a number of ways. There is a concern for Vitamin A toxicity in some people, but the Truth is that one would have to take so much vitamin A for an extended period of time before any toxicity would present. The real threat of it is practically nil, unless you have some preexisting condition making you predisposed to it.[66] By eating foods high in Vitamin A, we will also be ingesting trace elements found in real food that have not been identified yet. When eating natural foods as a source of vitamins and minerals, there are no reported cases of Vitamin A, or E toxicity, so it is always best to start eating real food, and don't rely solely on man-made products to get your nutrition.

In Summary...

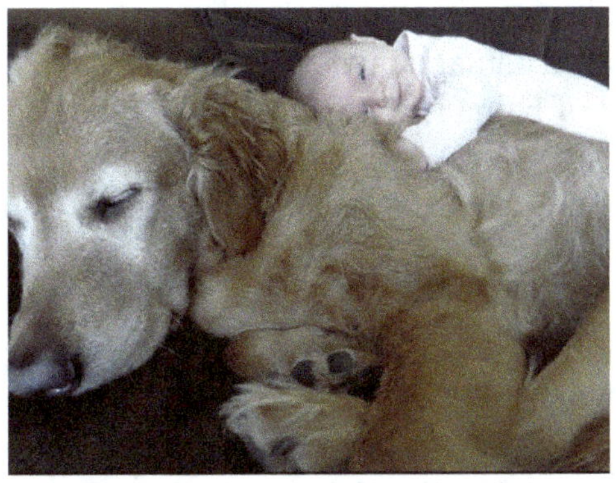

So as you can see, every single nutrient plays a part in restoring health and combating allergies. Since the typical diet in America is already lacking in so many of these ingredients, it is easy to see why allergies are so prevalent and more pervasive all the time. There is still more than can be said about diet and nutrition, but seeing how this is an eBook, written for the non-medical professional; Nutritional-Therapy is going to stop here.

In summary, the main effort in battling allergies should be focused on building up the body, so that it can process allergens, and not let them take over once they enter the body. Trying to manipulate the histamines with some man-made potion that only damages the liver and promises to keep you addicted to it for life is not the answer.

Adding supplements, building up your liver, adrenal glands, and intestinal bacteria will do far more to restore health than any medication will do. Medications will stop an urgent threat, and they have their place in society, but living on them will do far more damage than addressing the real problem of being able to combat allergens naturally.

If you make the decision to do what it takes to become healthy again, it is really very easy to do. All you have to do is make up your mind to do it. All these nutrients can be eaten with just a few supplements added to your existing diet.

Below is a brief summary of some of the items that should be included in your daily diet, and items that are easily bought at any nutrition center, or grocery store. Nothing here is dangerous in moderate amounts, and nothing here should contraindicate any existing medicines being taken, but it would be wise to check with your doctor if you have any pre-existing conditions.

While it is better to eat 5-6 small meals throughout the day, nutrition can be eaten in 1 meal, and last throughout the day. At the _very least_; an adult should add the following food to their diet until complete allergen tolerance is found. Remember, these supplements are naturally occurring in a normal diet, so there is no chance of overdosing.

- 1 to 3 bottles of vitamin water that includes all the B- vitamins
- 1 to 5 grams of Vitamin C daily
- 1 to 3 tablespoon of wheat germ daily
- A source of intestinal bacteria such as yogurt with live, active culture; or if yogurt can't be tolerated, substitute with acidophilus milk
- A reputable multi-vitamin such as General Nutrition Center's (GNC) Mega-Men or Mega-Woman
- Every effort should be made to eat high protein foods such as meats, fish, poultry, cheese, eggs, yogurt, milk, and fresh fruits and veggies. If this just sounds too foreign to you, start by adding 1-2 protein shakes to your daily diet instead. If you can eat these, you will be back on track in very little time.

If *food allergies* are already present, add these supplemental vitamins first, and then foods slowly in order to build up a tolerance to them before making any drastic changes. If your allergies are food related, then by all means speak with your physician before you reintroduce a known allergen. It would be a good idea to find a doctor who is educated in diet and nutrition, and then follow their advice- it is not enough to just understand it yourself.

With so many choices available in the market these days, it can be difficult to make the right decisions on what to eat. If you can remember to stay away from processed foods, and lean towards fresh fruit and vegetables, you will find many health issues fade away in a relatively short amount of time. By adding nutritional supplements, you will also be fine tuning your taste buds so that you will start to develop a taste for fresh food again.

It is not always easy, but nothing good ever is. However, if you are serious about eliminating allergies once and for all, then take this advice to heart. You will be outside, playing with the neighbors' pets, and enjoying all foods out in the spring time air in a very short time.

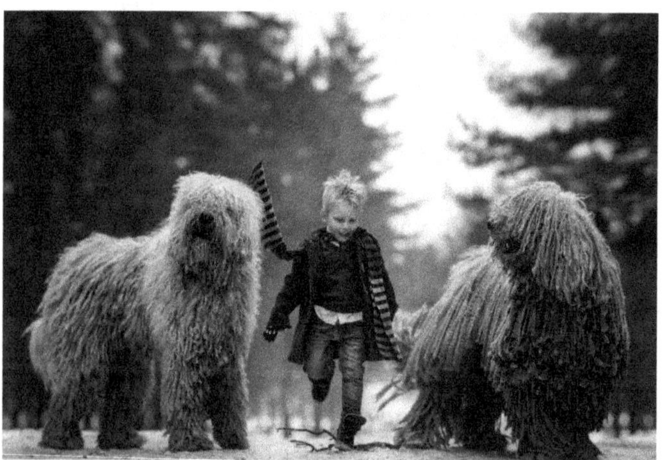

LIVE AGAIN!

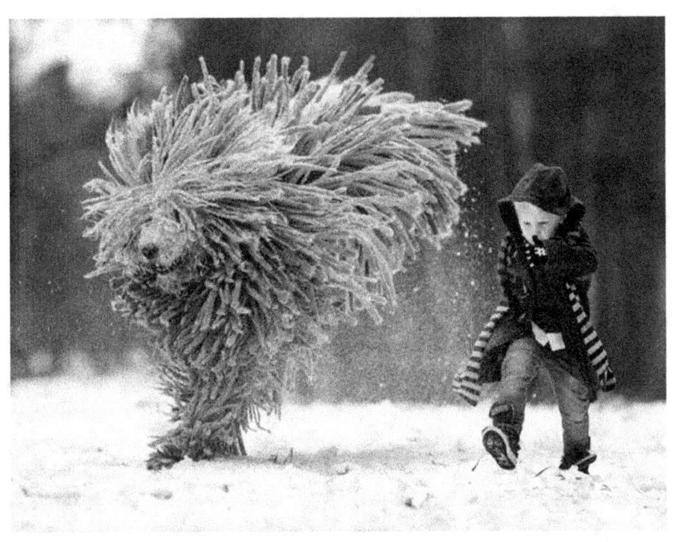

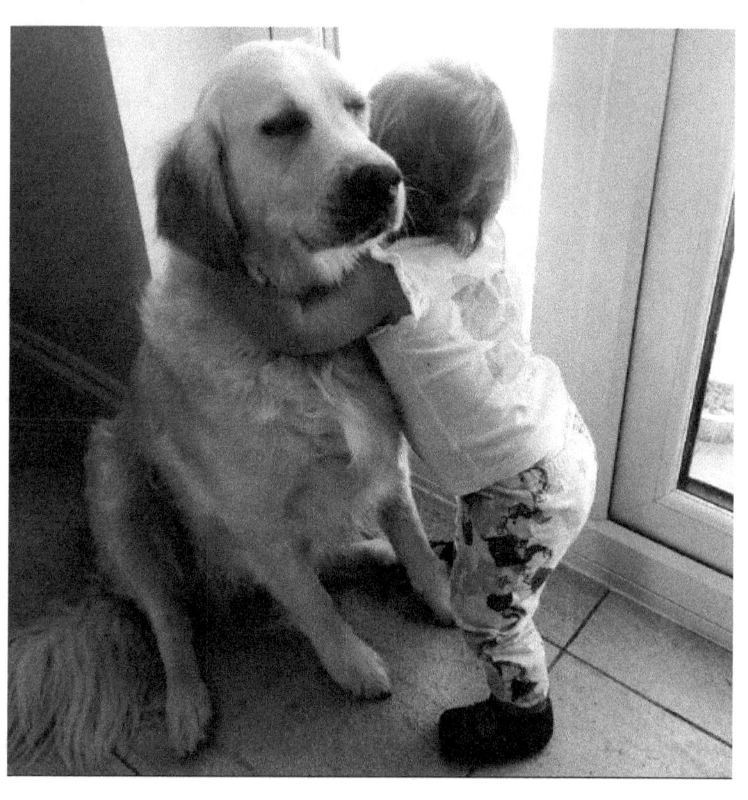

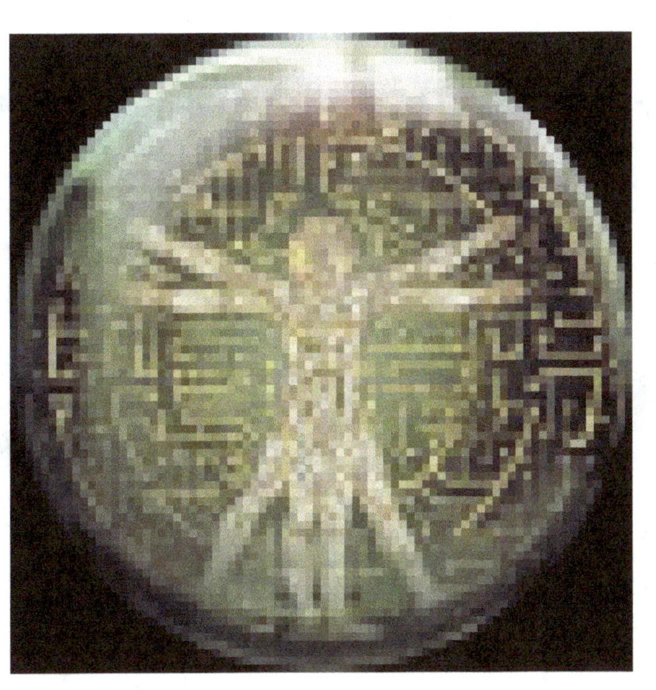

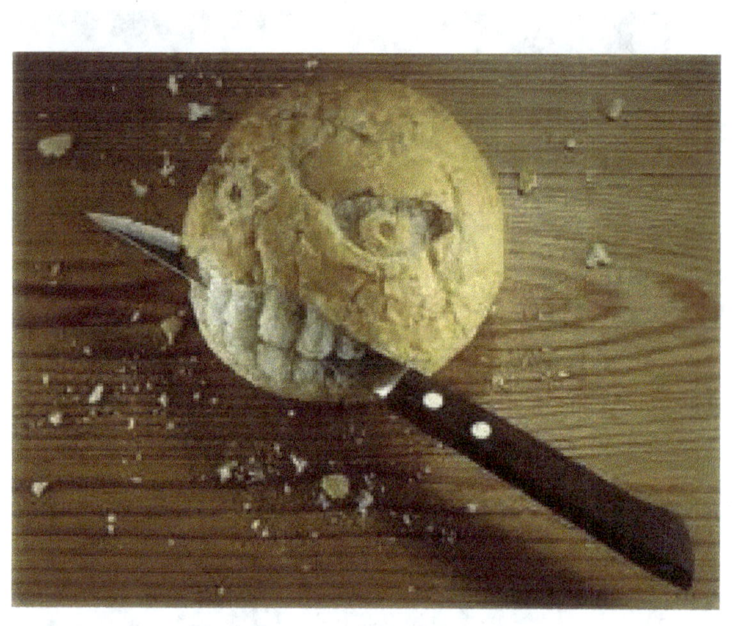

More Information Can Be Found At;

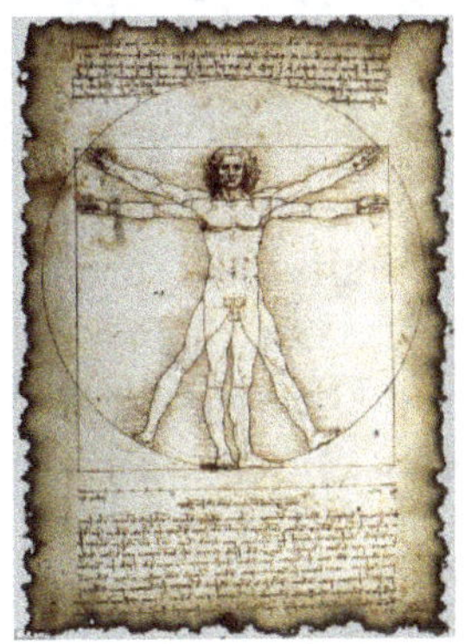

To find out more about treating your health with Nutrition, visit

https://www.nutritional-therapy.us/

Kerri Ryan
https://www.nutritional-therapy.us/
NutritionalTherapyUS@gmail.com

Alternative Medicine's Medical Disclaimer

The information on this site is not intended to be a substitute for professional medical advice, diagnosis or treatment. Each individual person has their own unique set of medical needs, and all information gathered here should be considered along with the advice of the reader's doctor. This information is intended to offer alternatives to traditional, drug related medical therapies, and the readers assume all responsibility when putting this information into effect. This information is accurate and true to the best of all authors' authority; is taken from numerous medical sources and referenced whenever possible. All content, including text, graphics, images and information, contained on or available through this publication is for general information purposes and does not take into account any other preexisting conditions. Readers will not hold ALTERNATIVE MEDICINE'S authors or administrators responsible for any adverse results.

NEVER DISREGARD PROFESSIONAL MEDICAL TREATMENT BECAUSE OF SOMETHING YOU HAVE READ ON OR ACCESSED THROUGH THIS MATERIAL.

Nutritional-Therapy will not be responsible or liable for any course of treatment, diagnosis, or any other information, services or products that are obtained through this publication; but rather offer alternatives to those wanting to get away from prescription drugs; and those wanting to restore health naturally without them.

For more information, please contact
NutritionalTherapyUS@gmail.com

You are encouraged to report negative side effects of prescription drugs to the FDA. Visit the FDA MedWatch website;
http://www.fda.gov/Safety/MedWatch/HowToReport/default.htm or call 1-800-FDA-1088 to find out more.

[1]
http://www.wrightslaw.com/info/section504.ada.peer.htmhttp://www.ncld.org/images/stories/Publications/AdvocacyBriefs/UnderstandingADAAA-Section504/UnderstandingADAAA-Section504.pdf

[2] http://download.journals.elsevierhealth.com/pdfs/journals/0022-3476/PIIS0022347610007870.pdf

[3] https://www.bustle.com/p/7-unexpected-potentially-dangerous-side-effects-of-taking-allergy-medicine-long-term-8970194

[4] https://www.bustle.com/profile/carina-wolff-1911169

[5] http://en.wikipedia.org/wiki/Allergen_immunotherapy

[6] http://en.wikipedia.org/wiki/Sublingual_immunotherapy

[7] http://en.wikipedia.org/wiki/Sublingual_immunotherapy

[8] http://www.amazon.com/Kerri-Ryan/e/B006P0FZUE/ref=ntt_athr_dp_pel_1

[9] http://www.stopmandatoryvaccination.com/vaccine-dangers/

[10] https://www.merriam-webster.com/dictionary/metabolic

[11] Selye, H., The Stress of Life, McGraw-Hill, New York, 1956; Selye, H., Candian Med. Journ. 61, 553, 1949

[12] Selye, H., Candian Med. Journ. 61, 553, 1949; Selye, H., The Stress of Life, McGraw-Hill, New York, 1956

[13] Pottenger, F.M., et al, Ann. West. Med. Surg. 6,484,1952; Tui, C., J. Clin. Nutrition, 1, 232, 1953; Goldfarb, A.A., et al, NY State J. Med. 61,2721, 1961

[14] Annand, J.C.,Practitioner, 175, 745, 1955; Moll, H.H., Brit. Med. J., 1, 976,1934; Simon, S.W., J. Allergy 22, 183, 1951

[15] Williams, R.J., Biochemical Individuality, Wiley, NY, 1956; Seronde, J., et al, J. Infectious Dis., 97, 35, 1955

[16] https://en.wikipedia.org/wiki/Thiamine_deficiency

[17] https://en.wikipedia.org/wiki/Pellagra

[18] http://en.wikipedia.org/wiki/Enriched_flour ; http://www.accessdata.fda.gov/scripts/cdrh/cfdocs/cfcfr/CFRSearch.cfm?fr=136.115;

[19] http://en.wikipedia.org/wiki/White_bread

[20] http://en.wikipedia.org/wiki/Enriched_flour ; http://en.wikipedia.org/wiki/Pellagra

[21]Williams, R.J., Biochemical Individuality, Wiley, NY, 1956; Seronde, J., et al, J. Infectious Dis., 97, 35, 1955

[22] http://www.livestrong.com/article/2707-facts-health-benefits-wheat-germ/

[23] Smith, L.W., et al, Antibiotic Med. Clin. Therap. 4, 515, 1957

[24] http://nutritiondata.self.com/topics/processing

[25] Irvine, W.T., Lancet, 1, 1064 and 1061, 1959; Epps, H.M.R., Biochem. J., 39,42, 1945; Wilson, C.W.M., J. Physiol. 125, 534, 1954

[26] Kaplan, H., et al, Ann. Allergy, 21,41,1963; Selye, H., The Stress of Life, McGraw-Hill, New York, 1956

[27] Cooper, L.F., et al, Nutrition in health and Disease, Lippincott, Phil., PA, 1958, ch. 26

[28] Vilter, R.W., et al, J. Lab. Clin. Med., 42,335,1953

[29] Cooper, L.F., et al, Nutrition in health and Disease, Lippincott, Phil., PA, 1958, ch. 26

[30] Irvine, W.T., Lancet, 1, 1064 and 1061, 1959; Mitchell, R.G. et al, J. Applied Physiol., 6, 387, 1954

[31] Irvine, W.T., Lancet, 1, 1064 and 1061, 1959; Sircus, W., Quart. J. Exp. Physiol., 38,25, 1953; Kaplan, H., et al, Ann. Allergy, 21,41,1963

[32] Selye, H., The Stress of Life, McGraw-Hill, New York, 1956; Kaplan, H., et al, Ann. Allergy 21, 41, 1963

[33] http://www.sciencedaily.com/releases/2007/04/070411170842.htm

[34] http://nutritiondata.self.com/topics/processing

[35] http://lpi.oregonstate.edu/infocenter/vitamins/pa/

[36] http://en.wikipedia.org/wiki/Pantothenic_acid

[37] Williams, R.J., Biochemical Individuality, Wiley, NY, 1956

[38] Williams, R.J., Biochemical Individuality, Wiley, NY, 1956; Seronde, J., et al, J. Infectious Dis., 97, 35, 1955

[39] http://www.anyvitamins.com/vitamin-b5-pantothenic-info.htm

[40] http://www.anyvitamins.com/vitamin-b5-pantothenic-info.htm; Selye, H., The Stress of Life, McGraw-Hill, New York, 1956

[41] Selye, H., The Stress of Life, McGraw-Hill, New York, 1956; Ershoff, B.H., et al, J. of Nutrition, 50, 299, 1953; Pudelkewicz, C., et al, J. of Nutrition, 70, 348, 1960

[42] Pottenger, F.M., et al, Ann. West. Med. Surg., 6, 484, 1952; Smith, L.W., et al, Antibiotic Med. Clin. Therapy, 4, 515, 1957

[43] http://www.nobelprize.org/nobel_prizes/medicine/laureates/1950/kendall-lecture.pdf

[44] Bicknell, F., and Prescott, F., The Vitamins in Medicine, Lee Found. For Nutritional Research, Mil. Wis., 1953

[45] http://www.mayoclinic.org/symptoms/eosinophilia/basics/definition/sym-20050752

[46] Vilter, R.W., et al, J. Lab. Clin. Med., 42,335,1953

[47] Vilter, R.W., et al, J. Lab. Clin. Med., 42,335,1953

[48] Pottenger, F.M., et al, Ann. West. Med. Surg., 6, 484, 1952; Smith, L.W., et al, Antibiotic Med. Clin. Therapy, 4, 515, 1957

[49] http://en.wikipedia.org/wiki/Linus_Pauling

[50] https://www.nobelprize.org/search/?query=linus+pauling

[51] Nutritional Review, 4, 259, 1946; Nutritional Review, 6, 215, 1948; Nutritional Review, 15, 185, 1957

[52] http://freehealthandbeautysecrets.com/?page_id=14

[53] Nutritional Review, 4, 259, 1946; Nutritional Review, 6, 215, 1948; Nutritional Review, 15, 185, 1957

[54] Bicknell, F., and Prescott, F., The Vitamins in Medicine, Lee Foundation For Nutritional Research, Mil., Wis., 1953

[55] Brown, E.A., et al, Ann. Allergy 7,1, 1949

[56] Bicknell, F., and Prescott, F., The Vitamins in Medicine, Lee Foundation For Nutritional Research, Mil., Wis., 1953; Klenner, F.R., Tri State Med. J. July 1954

[57] http://lpi.oregonstate.edu/mic/health-disease/skin-health/vitamin-C

[58] http://www.vitamincfoundation.org/collagen.html

[59] http://en.wikipedia.org/wiki/Vitamin_C#Collagen.2C_carnitine.2C_and_tyrosine_synthesis.2C_and_microsomal_metabolism

[60] http://www.vitamincfoundation.org/collagen.html

[61] http://www.amazon.com/Good-Cholesterol-Without-Drugs-ebook/dp/B006M60R40/ref=sr_1_1?ie=UTF8&qid=1347477785&sr=8-1&keywords=kerri+ryan+cholesterol

[62] http://en.wikipedia.org/wiki/Essential_fatty_acids

[63] http://www.todaysdietitian.com/newarchives/062909p48.shtml

[64] http://www.jbc.org/content/134/2/535.full.pdf

[65] http://www.boost-immune-health.com/mucushealth.html

[66] http://www.mayoclinic.org/drugs-supplements/vitamin-a/safety/hrb-20060201

Allergies are not permanent, and drugs are not the only way to treat them. The allergic reaction is simply the body's inability to process histamines that enter the body. Once you learn how to get the body to do this, you will not have any more allergies, no matter where they come from; pets, plants, foods or anything else.

Getting the body to address histamines, can be done through the addition of specific nutritional supplements that anyone of any age can take, and that won't interfere with any medications someone might be taking.

Learn the truth about allergies, and get yourself drug free once and for all.